Pulmonary Arterial Hypertension

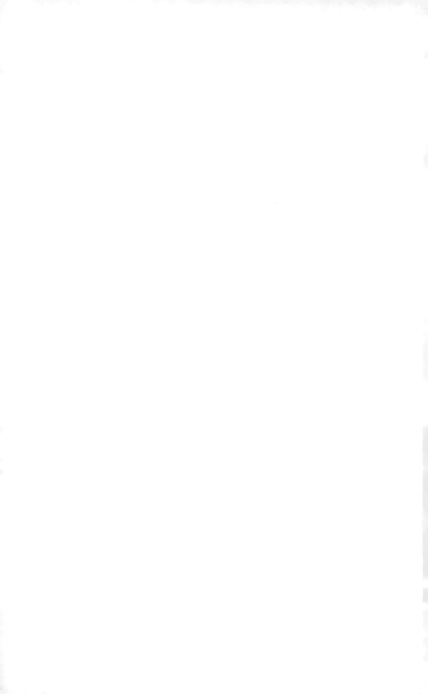

A Clinician's Guide to Pulmonary Arterial Hypertension

Simon Stewart PhD, FESC, FAHA, FCSANZ
Professor and Head of Preventative Cardiology,
Baker Heart Research Institute,
Melbourne, Australia

and

Geoff Strange RN BN
Regional Medical Manager,
Actelion Pharmaceuticals Asia-Pacific

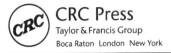

CRC Press
Taylor & Francis Group
Boca Raton London New York

CRC Press is an imprint of the
Taylor & Francis Group, an **informa** business

First published in the United Kingdom in 2007 by Informa Healthcare, Telephone House, 69–77 Paul St, London EC2A 4LQ. Informa Healthcare is a trading division of Informa UK Ltd. Registered Office: 37/41 Mortimer Street, London W1T 3JH. Registered in England and Wales Number 1072954.

Tel.: +44 (0)20 7017 6000
Fax.: +44 (0)20 7017 6699
Website: www.informahealthcare.com

Although every effort has been made to ensure that all owners of copyright material have been acknowledged in this publication, we would be glad to acknowledge in subsequent reprints or editions any omissions brought to our attention.

Although every effort has been made to ensure that drug doses and other information are presented accurately in this publication, the ultimate responsibility rests with the prescribing physician. Neither the publishers nor the authors can be held responsible for errors or for any consequences arising from the use of information contained herein. For detailed prescribing information or instructions on the use of any product or procedure discussed herein, please consult the prescribing information or instructional material issued by the manufacturer.

A CIP record for this book is available from the British Library.
Library of Congress Cataloging-in-Publication Data

Data available on application

ISBN 10: 1 84184 665 1
ISBN 13: 978 1 84184 665 1

Distributed in North and South America by
Taylor & Francis
6000 Broken Sound Parkway, NW (Suite 300)
Boca Raton, FL 33487, USA

Within Continental USA
Tel: 1(800)272 7737; Fax: 1(800)374 3401
Outside Continental USA
Tel: (561)994 0555; Fax: (561)361 6018
E-mail: orders@crcpress.com

Distributed in the rest of the world by
Thomson Publishing Services
Cheriton House
North Way
Andover, Hampshire SP10 5BE, UK
Tel.: +44 (0)1264 332424
E-mail: tps.tandfsalesorder@thomson.com

Composition by C&M Digitals (P) Ltd, Chennai, India

Contents

Preface

Pulmonary arterial hypertension, an uncommon but all too frequently fatal condition, represents one of those niche areas of medicine that attracts a small but fanatical following of experts. Such fanaticism is matched by the pharmaceutical companies who are able to leverage enormous profits from the successful treatment from a relatively small number of treated patients. It would be easy to become cynical about the symbiotic relationship between the experts and industry in pulmonary arterial hypertension but for one thing – improved awareness and treatment, leading to better health outcomes for those unfortunate (predominantly young women) to be affected.

As an 'outsider' who dabbled on the edges of pulmonary arterial hypertension, I have been more than fortunate to meet and talk to many of the experts who have put pulmonary arterial hypertension on the map and pioneered the significant therapeutic strides outlined in this book and its first incarnation (Simon Stewart, *Pulmonary Arterial Hypertension: A Pocketbook Guide* (2005), Taylor & Francis, London & New York). In publishing this new improved version of the book, I have been able to correct one important injustice done to one of the 'hidden' experts in pulmonary arterial hypertension – my co-author Geoff Strange. Suffering from his links to the pharmaceutical industry, Geoff was unwilling to come on board as a co-author of the first book; even though he richly deserved this position given his expert and impartial contribution. Thanks to the success of the first book, I'm delighted that we now have the opportunity to publish a second book that recognizes his expertise and co-authorship!

My aim in initiating and (co-)writing these two books was very simple: to introduce the wider health community to the importance of detecting potentially hidden pulmonary arterial hypertension and sending those unfortunate to be affected into the fanatical and passionate care routinely offered by expert centres. It is only through a united effort between the wider health community and the experts that we can positively alter the still fatal natural history of pulmonary arterial hypertension.

I hope this book achieves its aim and provides you with a succinct and invaluable overview of pulmonary arterial hypertension. Perhaps, one day, it will prompt you to suspect the presence of pulmonary arterial hypertension and save the life of an individual who would die prematurely without expert care and treatment.

Simon Stewart

Introduction

A relatively rare but devastating disease

Pulmonary arterial hypertension (PAH) is a relatively rare but potentially life-threatening disease. PAH is a particularly sinister condition that is, in most forms, likely to be diagnosed late and is associated with progressive clinical deterioration and premature death.[1-3]

The underlying processes that lead to the development of PAH are complex and the disease remains clinically silent until the right side of the heart begins to fail, initially only on exertion, but in later stages of the disease, at rest. Definitive diagnosis requires specialist skills. Invasive diagnostic procedures are necessary to determine the underlying aetiology and associated disease states. Due to the non-specific nature of the early symptom manifestations, diagnosis is typically not confirmed until up to 3 years from the initial symptom presentation, when disease pathophysiology is well developed.[1-3]

In recent years there has been increasing interest in the causes, consequences, and treatment of PAH. Pulmonary hypertension (PH) is defined haemodynamically as a mean pulmonary arterial pressure of >25 mmHg at rest or 30 mmHg with exercise.[2] PAH is specifically diagnosed by excluding other causes of PH, particularly left heart disease. Historically, much attention focussed on idiopathic and familial PAH (formerly known as primary PAH).[1-4] However, the contemporary view of PAH now recognizes a broader variety of aetiologies and associated conditions that may be targeted by PAH-specific therapies.[1]

This broadened view of PAH has highlighted a number of clinical quandaries in relation to its detection, diagnosis, and management. It has also stimulated the development and application of more effective treatment strategies to limit morbidity, improve quality of life, and prolong survival.

Without treatment, the prognosis for patients with significant PAH is poor.[5] Historically, the reported median life expectancy of those with idiopathic PAH in the era prior to PAH-specific treatments (see Chapter 5) was 2.8 years from diagnosis.[5] Similarly, 2-year survival rates in PAH associated with collagen vascular disease were reported to be as low as 40–55%[6] and PAH is a leading cause of death in individuals with PAH complicating systemic sclerosis.[7,8] Contemporary reports from France[9] and Scotland[10] have underlined the potential prognostic impact of a new era in PAH-specific management.

The prevailing view of PAH as an uncommon disease was based on reports that primary PAH (now known as idiopathic PAH) generated 1–2 incident cases per million per annum in the USA.[11] Similarly, reports of incidence rates for PAH related to congenital heart disease,[12] collagen vascular disease,[7,8] and other miscellaneous conditions, including HIV infection[13] and portal hypertension,[14] were slightly higher.[1,2] More recent data from the French National Registry of expert PAH Centres[9] and whole population data from Scotland[15] indicate that PAH is more likely a 'relatively rare' condition, with a prevalence ranging from 15 to 50 cases per million adults.

Given the rapid and expanding interest in the detection and management of PAH, particularly with the availability of more effective treatments, it is increasingly important for clinicians to be able to recognize this condition and direct patients to centres with experience in its assessment and treatment. Recognizing the potential for PAH in patients with a suspicious clinical profile is only the first step. In order to substantially improve health outcomes associated with such a difficult and heterogeneous condition, it is important for each health care system to have a clear and practical framework to facilitate the following:

- Identification of potential cases of PAH in a cost-efficient manner
- Rapid and accurate diagnosis of PAH and any underlying conditions that will determine treatment and overall management
- Application of effective treatments likely to improve the quality of life, functional status, and prognosis of affected patients.

An important step in this process has been the widespread adoption of the new classification system for PH and specifically PAH first developed by the World Health Organization (WHO) in 1998 and recently modified in 2003.[1] In parallel to this process has been the development and publication of expert guidelines in Europe[16] and North America.[17,18]

It is clear that responsibility for attaining the best possible health outcomes in this group of patients lies beyond experts in the disease (who have traditionally resided in Centres of Excellence in PAH) and extends to clinicians of all specialities and health professions who see many difficult and unusual cases in their clinical practice.

Aims of this book

This clinician's guide to PAH is designed to address several aims (Box 1.1).

Box 1.1   *Aims of this clinician's guide to PAH*

- Enhance the overall 'PAH awareness' of the wider clinical community.

- Facilitate an understanding of the epidemiology, pathophysiology, and clinical profile of PAH.

- Emphasize the need for active screening of high-risk patients and outline the screening and diagnostic process of identifying PAH.

- Outline the range and effectiveness of treatment options once PAH has been definitively diagnosed.

- Encourage the utilization of Centres of PAH Excellence.

- Promote a more collaborative and proactive model of health care to improve PAH-related health outcomes.

Additional PAH resources

This clinician's guide to PAH does not contain definitive and exhaustive information concerning PAH. Instead, it attempts to encapsulate the most important aspects of its detection and management. To assist those clinicians in search of more definitive information, an Appendix lists some of the most useful websites relating to PAH. Each chapter cites the most relevant and contemporary references, which are listed at the back of the book.

Disease background and epidemiology of pulmonary arterial hypertension

Definition of pulmonary arterial hypertension

In normal circumstances, resting pulmonary artery systolic pressure ranges from 18 to 25 mmHg (mean pulmonary artery pressures 12–16 mmHg). Pulmonary circulation, therefore, usually operates within a 'low resistance' environment and any increase in pulmonary vascular resistance leads to pulmonary hypertension. Pulmonary arterial hypertension is defined as a mean pulmonary artery pressure >25 mmHg at rest or >30 mmHg with exercise. The severity of PAH can be further delineated on the basis of this pressure (Box 2.1).

Box 2.1   Severity of PAH

- ■ Mild: 25–45 mmHg
- ■ Moderate: 46–65 mmHg
- ■ Severe: >65 mmHg

There are many potential causes of PAH and it therefore represents a heterogeneous clinical phenomenon that requires further elucidation to ensure appropriate screening, diagnosis, and management (Figure 2.1).[16–18]

Diagnostic classification

In order to facilitate the detection, diagnosis, and treatment of the many forms of pulmonary hypertension, including PAH, the WHO sponsored an expert consensus conference in Evian, in 1998 where a formal classification system was formulated. This system was recently updated and published following an expert meeting in Venice, in 2003.[1]

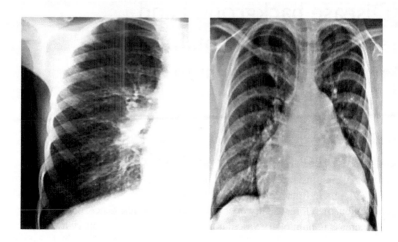

Figure 2.1 *Chest radiography suggestive of underlying PAH. The chest X-ray of affected individuals may show prominence of the main pulmonary artery, cardiomegaly, enlarged hilar vessels, and diminished peripheral vessels due to chronically increased pulmonary pressure.*

NB. Although up to 85% of patients with PAH develop an abnormal chest X-ray or 12-lead electrocardiograph (ECG), definitive assessment of pulmonary pressure is required for diagnosis of PAH (see Chapter 4).[16]

Table 2.1 shows the current classification system used to categorize the various forms of PH and the specific subcategory of PAH. It is important to note that modifications in the nomenclature relating to PAH involved the replacement of the term primary pulmonary hypertension (PPH) in favour of idiopathic PAH, and the recognition of familial PAH as a separate category. In addition, PAH is recognized as being 'related to' rather than 'secondary to' coexisting diseases such as connective tissue disease, HIV infection, and portal hypertension. Changes to other categories of pulmonary hypertension clarify terminology rather than rearrange the whole classification system devised by the WHO working group in 1998.

Epidemiology

Given the inherent difficulty in detecting and providing a definitive diagnosis of PAH, it should come as no surprise that its true incidence and prevalence within the general population is unknown. Most data emanate from national

Table 2.1   *Clinical classifications of pulmonary hypertension*[1]

1. Pulmonary arterial hypertension (PAH)

- Idiopathic PAH
- Familial PAH

Related to:

- Connective tissues diseases
- HIV
- Drugs and toxins
- Portal hypertension
- Anorexigens
- Congenital heart disease (systemic to pulmonary shunts, e.g. Eisenmenger's syndrome)
- Persistent pulmonary hypertension of the newborn
- Significant venous and/or capillary involvement

2. Pulmonary hypertension with left heart disease

- Left-sided atrial or ventricular heart disease
- Left valvular disease

3. Pulmonary hypertension with lung disease and/or hypoxaemia

- Chronic obstructive pulmonary disease
- Interstitial lung disease
- Sleep disorder breathing
- Alveolar hyperventilation disorders
- Chronic exposure to high altitude
- Developmental abnormalities

4. Pulmonary hypertension due to chronic thrombotic and/or embolic disease

- Thromboembolic obstruction of the proximal pulmonary arteries
- Thromboembolic obstruction of the distal pulmonary arteries
- Non-thrombotic pulmonary embolism (e.g. tumour or parasitic)

5. Miscellaneous disorders affecting the pulmonary vasculature (e.g. sarcoidosis)

registries and clinical trials and patients most likely to gravitate towards specialist centres. It is highly unlikely that large-scale population studies will determine the true epidemiological profile of PAH and those patients lucky enough to reach a specialist centre may be the exception rather than the rule. When considering, for example, heart failure, specialist centres typically treat younger patients in whom a differential diagnosis is less clouded by concurrent disease states and there are more severe symptoms due to advanced progression of the underlying disease state. There is little reason to presume that PAH differs from the heart failure scenario, except that in PAH there is a preponderance of younger women as opposed to younger men.[9,10]

This does not invalidate the type of epidemiological data published to date; it merely emphasizes the need for clinicians to resist stereotyping patients and ignoring clinical indications that a middle-aged man, for example, has developed right heart failure secondary to undiagnosed idiopathic PAH.

Incidence

Idiopathic and familial PAH have been reported to generate 1–2 cases per million each year in the USA.[5] Other causes of PAH, most notably collagen vascular disease (e.g. systemic sclerosis)[7,8] and congenital abnormalities leading to systemic to pulmonary shunts (e.g. Eisenmenger's syndrome)[12,19–21] are reported to be associated with a similar incidence rate. Contemporary data from the National Registry of PAH Centres of Excellence in France are consistent with these early reports.[9]

However, recent data from the whole Scottish population (with supportive data from a PAH Centre of Excellence) suggest that the incidence of idiopathic/ familial PAH over the 16-year period 1986–2001 was 4 cases per million/ annum (3 and 4 cases per million/annum in men and women, respectively) in those aged 16–65 years.[15] The equivalent rates for PAH-associated connective tissue disorders and congenital abnormalities during this period ranged from 1 to 3.5 cases per million/annum, respectively, in that country. Although these data showed that incidence rates have remained fairly constant in this age group, they also show that an increasing number of older individuals (aged >65 years) are being diagnosed with PAH. Consistent with these data, contemporary reports from Australia[3] suggest that idiopathic PAH generates approximately 3–10 cases per million each year. Certainly, with an increased awareness of PAH and increased detection rates, the reported incidence of PAH has risen in the past decade.

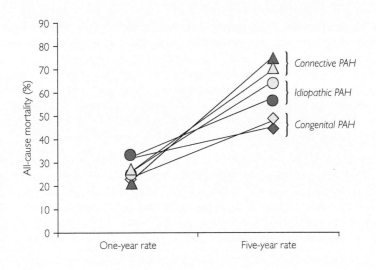

Figure 2.2 Actuarial 1- and 5-year case-fatality rates (men in red and women in yellow) related to PAH derived from Scottish population data (1986–2001). Figure adapted from original data.[10]

Prevalence

There are very few reports of the prevalence of PAH. However, given the rise in reported incident cases and improved survival rates, most probably due to the introduction of relatively effective treatment strategies (see Chapter 5), the underlying prevalence is most likely rising. In Scotland (total population 5 million), for example, the total number of surviving men and women aged 65 years or less being actively treated for idiopathic PAH, PAH related to scleroderma, and PAH related to congenital heart disease is reported to be 25, 15, and 12 cases per million per population.[15] The total point prevalence of these forms of PAH in Scotland in 2002 was 52 adult patients per million. Two-thirds of these cases are women and these estimates were confined to those aged < 65 years. Once again, these are likely to be underestimates of the true prevalence of PAH given that detected numbers of patients do not reflect the likely contribution of conditions such as connective tissue disorders.

Prognostic implications

Without treatment, the prognosis for patients with significant PAH is poor. Historically, the reported median life expectancy of those with idiopathic PAH in the era prior to PAH-specific treatments (see Chapter 5) was 2.8 years from diagnosis.[5] Similarly, 2-year survival rates in PAH associated with collagen vascular disease were reported to be as low as 40–55%[6] and PAH is a leading cause of death in individuals with PAH complicating systemic sclerosis.[7,8] Contemporary reports from France[9] and Scotland[10] have underlined the potential prognostic impact of a new era in PAH-specific management.

Recent whole population data from Scotland for the period 1986–2001 demonstrate that in the pre PAH-specific treatment era, mortality rates related to all forms of PAH were extremely high. For example, Figure 2.2 shows the 1- and 5-year actuarial survival rates associated with idiopathic, connective tissue, and congenital heart disease related PAH in hospitalized patients aged 16–65 years during this period.[15]

These data are derived from the linked Scottish Morbidity Record Scheme.[22] Largely consistent with data from the National Institute of Health in the USA, 1-year case fatality in those with PAH associated with collagen vascular disease was 25%, rising to 70% at 5 years. A comparison of the demographic profile of incident cases highlighted the fact that patients with connective tissue disorders are more likely to be screened for PAH and treated earlier. It should be noted, however, that patients with connective tissue-related PAH commonly have a worse prognosis than those with idiopathic PAH when presenting with the same haemodynamic profile.

A major limitation of population-derived data is the lack of specific detail collected concerning the progression of disease. As Figure 2.3 demonstrates, patients who exhibit more advanced symptomology, as determined by a more severe WHO classification (Class IV compared with Class II and III), have a markedly worse prognosis.[5] Overall, these data reinforce three important points in relation to PAH:

■ regardless of extent of disease progression and associated disease states, survival rates in PAH are poor
■ the potential for positive effects of new modalities of treatment is high
■ there is a strong possibility that earlier detection and proactive management of PAH will slow the typical disease progression/deterioration.[23]

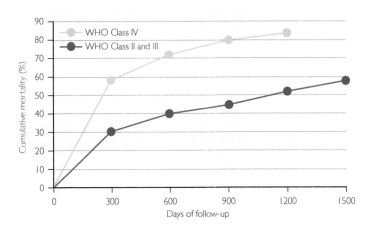

Figure 2.3 *Differential survival based on WHO Classification of PAH-related symptoms (Class II & III vs Class IV). Figure adapted from original data.*[5]

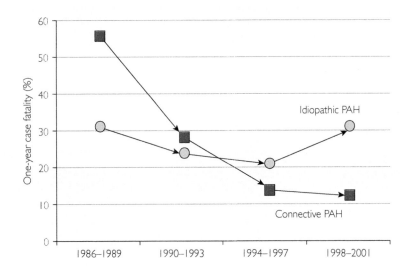

Figure 2.4 *Trends in 1-year actuarial survival in patients with idiopathic PAH or PAH related to a connective tissue disorder. Figure adapted from original data.*[10]

In support of the above clinical points and the importance of functional class and survival, Williams and colleagues demonstrated functional improvements and halving in the relative risk of dying associated with PAH-specific treatments in a cohort of patients with PAH related to connective tissue disorders.[23] Figure 2.4 shows historical improvements in the survival of the same type of hospitalized patients (aged 16–65 years) in Scotland.[10]

When combined with low PAH-related mortality rates recently reported from France,[9] these data emphasize the potential to dramatically improve survival rates via early detection and intervention with PAH-specific treatments.

Pulmonary arterial hypertension – increasing our understanding of disease pathophysiology

3

Introduction to the pathophysiology of PAH

Our understanding of the pathophysiology of PAH is still in its infancy, although significant advances have been made based on molecular science, genetics, and the understanding of the clinico-pathological interactions recognized in the WHO classification scheme. Undoubtedly, the pathophysiology of PAH is complex, pivoting around the concepts of vasoconstriction, vascular remodelling, and thrombosis. Vasoactive substances, growth factors, inflammatory mediators, and components of the clotting/coagulation system are all involved to varying degrees.[24] This complex interplay is only just being decoded, but already there have been both real and potential therapeutic targets unearthed.

This chapter will discuss some of the underlying mechanisms and mediators responsible for (or associated with) the development of PAH, and how these interact to cause the problems encountered in clinical practice.

Vascular wall remodelling/vasconstriction and platelet activation

Mechanisms

Postmortem studies of PAH typically show histopathological changes in pulmonary resistance arteries, characterized by marked obstructive lesions.[25–27] These lesions represent proliferation of endothelial and smooth muscle cells and are the hallmark of PAH.[28] They cause progressive occlusion of the vessel lumen and provide an obvious reason for the development of PAH (see Figure 3.1). These lesions also highlight the fact that definitive treatments for

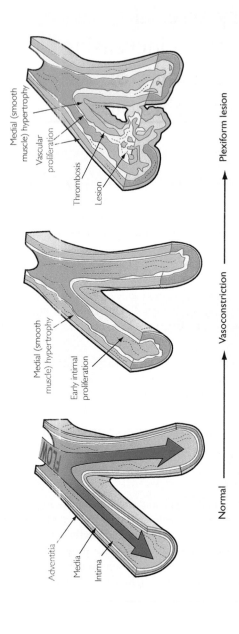

Figure 3.1 Developing obstructive plexiform lesions in pulmonary arteries.

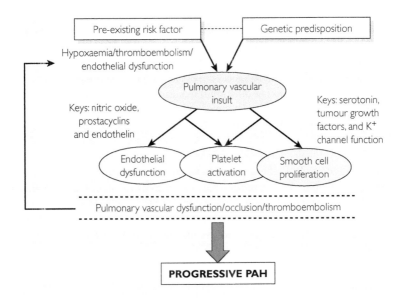

Figure 3.2 Algorithm of the pathophysiology of PAH.

PAH will require agents with antiproliferative and/or remodelling potential, as opposed to pure vasodilator treatments.[29,30] Reinforcing the importance of these lesions and potential therapeutic strategies, this process has been recently described as tumour-like in its development.[30] PAH can, however, develop in the absence of these distinct lesions in the pulmonary vasculature. In this setting, it is likely there are diffuse changes in the structure of pulmonary resistance arteries, in addition to altered vasoreactivity (provoking vasoconstriction) and increased platelet activation (leading to thromboembolism) leading to progressive PAH.[31,32]

Figure 3.2 represents an algorithm demonstrating how all three key components of PAH (vasoconstriction, vascular wall remodelling, and platelet activation/aggregation) have the potential to form a pathological triad that may lead to a cascade of vascular dysfunction, increasing pulmonary vascular resistance and progressive clinical deterioration. Standard pharmacological treatment of PAH (see Chapter 5) aims to interrupt this pathological cascade.

Vasoreactivity

Normal resting (pulmonary) arterial tone is maintained by a balance of endogenous vasodilators and vasoconstrictors. Studies of PAH have shown that an imbalance on either side can lead to the development of pulmonary hypertension. In addition, many of these endogenous substances not only affect resting vascular tone (vasoconstriction or dilatation) but also have effects on cell (especially smooth muscle) proliferation, platelet aggregation, and vascular remodelling. For example, levels of nitric oxide (NO) and prostacyclin are diminished in PAH.[28,29,33–35] Nitric oxide and prostacyclin are both potent endogenous vasodilators. Prostacyclin also has potent antiplatelet effects and inhibits smooth muscle cell proliferation. Both these agents have proven to be effective treatments for PAH – see Chapter 5.[34,36] Conversely, vasoconstrictors such as endothelin and thromboxane are present in increased concentrations in pulmonary hypertension. Endothelin, in particular, has potent proliferative effects. Thus, endothelin provides an attractive target for effective therapy in PAH.[35,37–43]

Endothelin

Endothelin is a potent and long-lasting vasoconstrictor that is 100 times more potent than noradrenaline (norepinephrine).[38] In addition to being a potent vasoconstrictor, it is directly associated with fibrosis (predominantly mediated via the ET_B receptor), vascular cell hypertrophy, inflammation, and neurohormonal activation.[44,45] Its synthesis is triggered by numerous factors, including localized mediators such as inflammatory cytokines, and extrinsic factors such as low oxygen tension and increased arterial wall shear stress (e.g. in the presence of an obstructive plexiform lesion in the pulmonary vasculature).[45,46] The elevation of both plasma and tissue endothelin levels, and increased expression of endothelin receptors, are seen in pathological conditions such as PAH, acute and chronic heart failure, cardiogenic shock, acute coronary syndromes, and fibrotic lung disease.[47] Its role in connective tissue diseases is well documented, with evidence suggesting that elevated endothelin levels contribute to the vascular and fibrotic manifestations characteristic of systemic sclerosis.[48]

High plasma endothelin levels have been shown to correlate not only with severity of disease but also with prognosis for patients with both idiopathic PAH and that relating to connective tissue disease.[42,43] The growing evidence of the pathological role of endothelin in PAH has led to the development of endothelin receptor antagonists, such as bosentan, sitaxsentan, and ambrisentan, as a targeted therapeutic approach to disease pathogenesis.[35,49,50]

K+ channel function

Abnormal K+ channel function in pulmonary vascular smooth muscle also appears to be involved in the development of PAH. Hypoxia has been shown to selectively inhibit the function and expression of voltage-gated K+ channels in pulmonary arterial smooth muscle cells. Via this mechanism, acute hypoxia induces membrane depolarization, and a rise in cytosolic Ca^{2+} that triggers vasoconstriction. In addition, caspace activity is inhibited, resulting in an inhibition of apoptosis, and unchecked cell proliferation resulting in vascular remodelling.[51–53]

In addition to the above, it is useful to consider the way pulmonary hypertension is now classified to give us insights into the underlying pathophysiology. In part, this classification was born from an understanding of the different contributions of various disease states to the development of pulmonary hypertension, and PAH in particular.

The genetic basis of PAH

In the original (1998) WHO classification, familial PAH was thought of as a subsection of so-called primary pulmonary hypertension.[1] The latest classification, however, recognizing the identification and clarification of the gene responsible for familial PAH, classifies this as a separate entity.[10] Furthermore, it is known that the genetic defect(s) responsible for familial PAH is present in 10% of cases of idiopathic PAH.[4]

The gene defects identified as the cause of familial PAH are related to mutations in the bone morphogenetic protein receptor type 2 (BMPR2). This receptor and its ligand (bone morphogenetic protein 2) are part of the transforming growth factor beta (TGF-β) superfamily of signalling pathways. Normal activation of this receptor produces signals that inhibit proliferation, particularly of pulmonary artery smooth muscle cells. More than 40 BMPR2 gene mutations have been identified, and all lead to loss of this inhibition of cellular proliferation.[54–56]

In addition to the BMPR2 abnormalities, mutations in other genes have also been proposed as having a role in the development of pulmonary hypertension. Mutations in the ALK-1 receptor (activin-like kinase), also a member of the TGF-β family, have been linked to the development of PAH in patients suffering from hereditary haemorrhagic telangiectasia.[57] Likewise, genetic polymorphisms of the serotonin transporter (5-HTT) have been linked with PAH associated with hypoxia and fenfluramine use.[58] The role of these and other genetic abnormalities is providing a very fruitful area of research into both the pathogenic mechanisms underlying the development of PAH and the identification of potential therapeutic targets.

Systemic sclerosis (scleroderma)

Pulmonary hypertension is recognized as a lethal complication of all forms of systemic sclerosis. Endothelin has been postulated as having a pivotal role in the pathogenesis of the pulmonary vascular disease associated with this condition, which has all the hallmarks pathologically of PAH.[7,8,48] There are, however, significant clinical differences compared to other forms of PAH, relating principally to late presentation and/or recognition of the pulmonary vascular abnormality. This occurs in the main because of the significant co-morbidities associated with the underlying condition that often dominate the clinical presentation early in the disease. As a consequence, patients with systemic sclerosis often present in advanced stages of right ventricular dysfunction and functional decline, and, as a result, treatment outcomes are generally less satisfactory when compared to idiopathic PAH for example: although there is evidence that survival rates are improving in this group with the application of more specific PAH treatments.[10,23]

Pulmonary hypertension remains the most common cause of mortality in systemic sclerosis. Any patient with systemic sclerosis may present at any stage in their disease with vasculopathy, interstitial lung disease, or a combination of both.[59]

Other causes of PAH

As indicated in Table 2.1, portal hypertension,[14] human immunodeficiency virus (HIV) infection,[3,60] and anorectic agents[11,58] are external factors that can also lead to PAH. The use of appetite-suppressant drugs (amphetamine derivatives such as fenfluramine and dexfenfluramine) for more than 3 months is associated with a greater than 30-fold increased risk of developing pulmonary hypertension.[58] This complication has been linked to abnormal serotonin metabolism and polymorphisms in the serotonin transporter mechanism. The precise mechanisms by which portal hypertension and HIV infection lead to PAH are unknown.

Congenital abnormalities

Pulmonary vascular remodelling occurs in response to the shear stress caused by significant increases in pulmonary blood flow. This situation is most commonly encountered in congenital heart disease associated with systemic to pulmonary shunts.[20,21,61] The chronic increase in pulmonary blood flow leads to the development of PAH that is pathologically indistinguishable from idiopathic PAH. When the pulmonary arterial pressure exceeds systemic levels, reversal of the shunt occurs, with resultant cyanosis – Eisenmenger's syndrome.[19]

Persistent pulmonary hypertension of the newborn (PPHN) is a rare disorder of neonates. An elevated pulmonary vascular resistance is required for an effective fetal circulation; however, if this state persists after birth, pulmonary to systemic shunting occurs through persisting fetal channels (e.g. the ductus arteriosus), thereby bypassing the lungs and resulting in systemic arterial hypoxaemia.[20,33] As in many forms of PAH, the mechanisms underlying the development of pulmonary hypertension in this setting are poorly understood. The outcome of this condition, however, has been markedly improved with the use of inhaled nitric oxide therapy.

Pulmonary arterial hypertension – clinical profile and diagnosis

4

Clinical profile

It is important to remember that the key underlying haemodynamic factor in any form of PH is the increase in the pulmonary vascular resistance in response to the remodelled pulmonary circulation. The primary driver of this pathological process, therefore, is largely clinically silent until the response is manifested by changes (both acute and chronic) in right ventricular function. As such, without treatment, to relieve chronic PAH, particularly in its severest form, patients typically develop progressive right ventricular hypertrophy, dilatation, and associated right ventricular dysfunction – see Figure 4.1.[62–65] Without appropriate treatment, therefore, the right ventricle progressively fails, eventually resulting in death.

As indicated, many of the pathological changes associated with PAH may not produce significant and readily indentifiable symptoms until the disease has progressed significantly (i.e. when right heart failure has developed as a consequence of increased pulmonary vascular resistance). In addition, the clinical profile of PAH may also be obscured by the underlying disease state (e.g. systemic sclerosis), particularly where other factors have a detrimental effect on exercise tolerance.

Symptoms

The most common symptom of PAH is progressive exertional dyspnoea. Overall, a patient's description of the presenting symptoms is often vague and may lead to an alternative diagnosis (e.g. asthma). Depending on the stage of disease and degree of right ventricular compromise, patients can also present with symptoms such as:

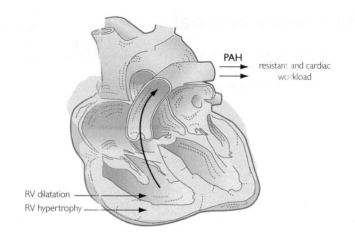

PAH

resistant and cardiac workload

RV dilatation

RV hypertrophy

Figure 4.1   *Right ventricular failure secondary to pulmonary arterial hypertension.*

- presyncope and syncope
- central chest pain
- fatigue
- palpitations
- cough and occasionally haemoptysis.

Signs

Physical examination is often normal in early stages of the disease process, with the classical signs of pulmonary hypertension only becoming evident as right ventricular hypertrophy and failure develop. The following signs are indicative of right ventricular hypertrophy or pre-established right heart failure secondary to chronic PAH:

- left parasternal systolic lift
- accentuated pulmonary valve closure sound (loud P2)
- tricuspid regurgitant murmur
- raised jugular venous pressure
- RV 3rd heart sound
- hepatomegaly
- peripheral oedema and ascites.

Clinical investigations

Diagnostic investigations are shown in Box 4.1.[66]

Box 4.1   Clinical investigations of PAH

Imaging:

- chest radiograph
- echocardiogram
- ventilation perfusion scan
- high-resolution computed tomography (CT) of the lungs.

Respiratory:

- arterial blood gases in room air
- lung function testing
- nocturnal oxygen saturation monitoring.

Cardiology:

- electrocardiography (ECG)
- six-minute walk test (6MWT)
- right heart catheterization.

Blood investigations:

- biochemistry and haematology
- thrombophilia screen
- human immunodeficiency virus (HIV).

Urine:

- β-hCG (beta-human chorionic gonadotrophin) – women.

Routine investigations will provide evidence suggesting the diagnosis of pulmonary hypertension. For example, Figure 4.2 shows the pattern of right ventricular 'strain' seen in the ECG of a patient with right ventricular hypertrophy secondary to PAH. The majority of patients with PAH have an abnormal ECG.[1] Similarly, a chest X-ray may show proximal pulmonary

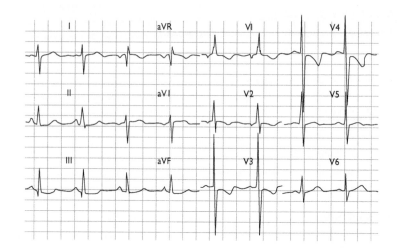

Figure 4.2 *12-lead ECG from a patient with right ventricular failure/hypertrophy secondary to PAH. Note the typical right ventricular strain pattern and right axis deviation, as denoted by positive R waves in leads V1, V2, and aVl.*

artery enlargement and/or cardiomegaly. Both 12-lead ECG and chest X-ray represent readily available screening tools for PAH (see Chapter 6), but it must be emphasized that both tests may be substantially normal in patients with symptomatic PAH, particularly in the earlier stages of the disease, but also occasionally in later disease stages.[66]

If pulmonary hypertension is suspected clinically, the next step is to evaluate the patient with transthoracic echocardiography. Doppler assessment of the right ventricular systolic pressure (RVSP), through measurement of the tricuspid regurgitant jet, gives an estimate of pulmonary artery pressure. In addition, there may be evidence of right ventricular hypertrophy and dysfunction.[67–70]

There is emerging evidence that stress echocardiography may be an appropriate strategy for case-finding patients at high risk of developing PAH (i.e. those with a connective tissue disorder).[70]

To confirm the diagnosis of PAH, raised left atrial pressure must be excluded by right heart catheter.[66] This procedure allows accurate measurement of pulmonary haemodynamics and determination of the patient's prognostic outlook.[65] Investigations used to either rule out PH or confirm associated pathology (e.g. pulmonary embolism) are further described in Chapter 6.

Clinical indicators of disease progression

There are a range of non-invasive and invasive indices/parameters used to monitor disease progression in PAH. The most commonly used of these are described below.

WHO functional class

As worsening dyspnoea on exertion is the most obvious and probably most sensitive marker of the underlying disease progression associated with PAH, it has proven to be the most practical means of delineating the clinical status of affected patients. As such, the WHO adopted the NYHA functional class (first applied to heart failure)[71] to stratify the clinical status of patients with PAH, and guide appropriate management according to their response/non-response to medical treatment (Table 4.1).

Patients whose clinical profile is consistent with WHO Class IV usually have signs of advanced right heart failure and there is little doubt that the progression from WHO Class I to IV mirrors the evolution/progression of right-sided heart failure secondary to the underlying PAH. As can be appreciated, patients in WHO Class I with underlying PAH are unlikely to be diagnosed unless investigated for another reason. Most patients present in WHO Class III and IV and have already developed right ventricular dysfunction.

Six-minute walk test

In addition to asking patients about their physical limitations and classifying their responses according to an agreed formula (e.g. WHO class), it is clearly desirable to gain a more objective measure of their functional capabilities. In this respect, the easiest, most tolerated and realistic test of a patient's ability to carry out activities of daily living is the 6-minute walk test (6MWT). This test is as simple as it sounds, only requiring an experienced supervisor to measure how far a patient can walk over a flat and unobstructed surface (32 metres in length) during the predefined time-frame of 6 minutes.[72,73] This simple walk test is sensitive to changes in cardiac function and can predict subsequent morbidity and mortality in PAH patients.[74] Like the WHO class, the results of this walk test may vary, so it is important to examine historical trends in patients rather than rely on a single test (i.e. using the patient as

Table 4.1 WHO functional classification of PAH[2]

WHO functional class	Symptomatic profile
Class I	Patients with pulmonary hypertension but without resulting limitation of physical activity. Ordinary physical activity does not cause undue dyspnoea or fatigue, chest pain, or near syncope
Class II	Patients with pulmonary hypertension resulting in slight limitation of physical activity. They are comfortable at rest. Ordinary physical activity causes undue dyspnoea or fatigue, chest pain, or near syncope
Class III	Patients with pulmonary hypertension resulting in marked limitation of physical activity. They are comfortable at rest. Less than ordinary activity causes undue dyspnoea or fatigue, chest pain, or near syncope
Class IV	Patients with pulmonary hypertension with inability to carry out any physical activity without symptoms. These patients manifest signs of right heart failure. Dyspnoea and/or fatigue may even be present at rest. Discomfort is increased by any physical activity

their own control following application of treatment). Improvements in right ventricular function with effective treatment can also be accurately monitored by 6MWT results. Data from this simple test can also be combined with that from the commonly used Borg dyspnoea index: a self-measure of perceived breathlessness.[75]

Haemodynamic parameters

If available, a number of haemodynamic parameters may be measured and provide concrete evidence of PAH and associative changes in cardiopulmonary function. The following parameters, often measured in Centres of

Clinical Excellence, are pivotal to determining a specific cause and diagnosis of PAH, with associated decisions relating to appropriate treatment and prognostic outlook:

- pulmonary artery pressure
- cardiac index
- pulmonary vascular resistance
- right atrial pressure
- pulmonary capillary wedge pressures.

It is important to note, of course, that the definitive diagnostic tool for PAH is right heart catheterization, providing a direct measure of pulmonary pressures.[66]

Respiratory function tests

These tests may include lung volumes and carbon monoxide (CO) diffusion capacity. Respiratory function tests often show a disproportionate reduction in carbon monoxide diffusion in the lung (DLCO – around 50% of predicted in moderate PAH), with at most a mild-to-moderate restrictive lung defect. The reduction in DLCO is greater than that seen with comparable symptomatic left heart failure and reflects the loss of effective or functioning pulmonary vasculature characteristic of PAH.[66] Pulmonary diffusing capacity may be clinically important in uncovering PAH in high-risk patient groups (e.g. those with connective tissue disorders).[59]

Improving outcomes in pulmonary arterial hypertension – pharmacological and surgical treatment strategies

5

The evolving treatment of PAH

To the uninitiated it may appear that there has always been a wealth of PAH-specific therapies available. However, it has only been in recent years that the therapeutic armoury to effectively manage PAH has dramatically increased; hence, historically poor survival rates. It was not until 1981 when heart–lung transplantation was introduced, that an effective treatment for PAH became available. Challenged by the limited number of organ donors, medical treatments have been sought, the most successful of which can now postpone the need for transplantation.

Increasing interest in PAH has led to many advances in treatment. The 3rd World Symposium on Pulmonary Arterial Hypertension (Venice 2003) represented a significant event in the clinical management of PAH. At this time, an expert task force was able to review clinical trial data to determine the clinical efficacy of a broad range of therapeutic strategies. A published report arising from this meeting[76] and subsequent expert guidelines published in Europe and North America,[16–18] now provide clinicians with a strong evidence base to manage patients with PAH.

Figure 5.1 synthesizes the latest expert advice published following the 2003 World Symposium[76] and the most recent North American guidelines.[18] In both cases, a grading system, based on the strength of clinical trial evidence for study design and efficacy, was applied to each treatment listed in this figure. Epoprostenol[77,78] bosentan,[79] inhaled iloprost,[80] and sildenafil[81] were all awarded the highest strengths of expert recommendation.[18,76] Importantly, in a rapidly evolving therapeutic environment the choice of first-line therapy for patients with symptomatic PAH now involves a combination of prostacyclin

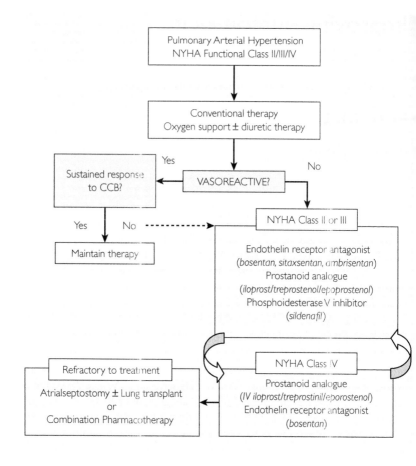

Figure 5.1 *A synthesis of current evidence-based guidelines for the management of pulmonary arterial hypertension.*[18,76] *CCB = calcium channel blocker, IV = intravenous.*

analogues, endothelin receptor antagonists, and phosphodiesterase type 5 inhibitors. In this context, choice of therapy takes into consideration, evidence, clinical judgement, regulatory approval, mode of administration, adverse event profile, cost, and patient preferences. The role and purpose of these treatments are overviewed, tabulated, and presented in more detail in Table 5.1.

Table 5.1 Overview of current treatment options for PAH*

Treatment	Indication	Contraindications	Comments
Anticoagulation: *warfarin*	Prevention of pulmonary arterial thrombosis	Caution in connective tissue disease	Associated with prolonged survival in idiopathic PAH.[63] There are no published data in other forms of PAH
Oxygen therapy	Patient with associated lung disease. Adult nocturnal desaturation (2 L/min)	May cause some vasoconstriction. Use with caution and closely monitor	Integral part of the management of all forms of pulmonary hypertension[1,124–127]
Supportive medical therapy: *diuretics, digoxin*	Presence of right heart failure. Digoxin may improve cardiac output in refractory patients	Digoxin used with caution in the elderly due to potential toxicity	Diuretics remain the gold standard for symptom relief of fluid overload in right heart failure.[128] ACE inhibitors and beta-blockers are superior to digoxin in other forms of heart failure[129]
Calcium antagonists: diltiazem, nifedipine, amlodipine	Reduction in pulmonary artery pressure (PAP). Reduction in mortality with sustained response. Patients with right ventricular impairment should be considered for	Calcium antagonists should *not* be started before an acute vasodilator study. Patients who do not respond to a vasodilator challenge would be unlikely to	A patient demonstrating an acute response to a vasodilator test is defined as a reduction in mPAP by at least 10 mmHg to at least <40 mmHg with a maintained or improved CO. A sustained response is reported in <10% of patients[84–86]

(Continued)

Table 5.1 (Continued)

Treatment	Indication	Contraindications	Comments
	amlodipine. Therapy should be initiated in hospital and carefully titrated according to blood pressure, oxygen saturations, and exercise tolerance	respond to calcium antagonists. CCBs should be avoided if cardiac Index (CI) is <2.1 l/min/m² and/or right atrial pressure (RAP) > ±10 mmHg	
Prostaglandin therapy: epoprostenol, iloprost, treprostinil (IV, SC, or inhaled)	Idiopathic PAH, familial PAH, and PAH associated with connective tissue disorders and a small number of inoperable CTEPH	Potential for rebound pulmonary hypertension if withdrawn suddenly. Dose titration is required. Continuous IV line and potential infections. Slight pain in SC form. Variable response in inhaled form between doses (see various product information for full list of contraindications)	IV epoprostenol associated with prolonged long-term survival, 6MWT, and haemodynamic improvements. Specialist care is required for complex and technically challenging therapy[90,92]

(Continued)

Table 5.1 (Continued)

Treatment	Indication	Contraindications	Comments
Endothelin receptor antagonists: *bosentan, sitaxsentan, ambrisentan*	Idiopathic PAH, familial PAH, PAH associated with connective tissue disorders, congenital heart disease, HIV/AIDS, and inoperable CTEPH	A class effect of potential elevations in liver enzymes (ALT/AST) (see various product information for full list of contraindications)	ERAs have been shown to improve symptoms, exercise capacity, and haemodynamics. Bosentan and ambrisentan have been shown to delay disease progression in reducing time to clinical worsening.[79,111] Bosentan has been shown to prolong survival[100]
Phosphodiesterase type 5 inhibitors: *sildenafil*	Idiopathic PAH, familial PAH, PAH associated with connective tissue disorders, and congenital heart disease	Caution as hypotension may occur in higher than the approved (20 mg tds) dose (see various product information for full list of contraindications)	The only available data on long-term response with sildenafil is in 80 mg tds. No long-term evidence is available on the currently approved dose (20 mg tds)[112]

*Please refer to product information and regulatory authority guidelines for each form of therapy. iPAH – Idiopathic PAH, CTD – Connective tissue disorder, CHD – Congenital Heart Disease, CTEPH – Chronic Thromboembolic pulmonary hypertension.

Medical management

The medical treatments summarized in Table 5.1 that form part of the gold standard management of PAH are principally designed to directly improve right ventricular function (primarily by reducing cardiac afterload by addressing the pulmonary vascular resistance (PVR) to flow),thereby acting to ameliorate underlying pulmonary hypertension and reduce thromboembolic load.

Basic care of patients with pulmonary hypertension

All patients with pulmonary hypertension and right ventricular dysfunction, regardless of the cause, require standard therapy with diuretics (to reduce right ventricular preload), antiarrhythmic agents such as digoxin and/or amiodarone (to maintain sinus rhythm wherever possible)[82] and warfarin. Warfarin therapy has been shown to improve survival rates in those with idiopathic PAH.[63] Calcium antagonists (e.g. diltiazem and nifedipine) have been shown to be effective in reducing pulmonary arterial pressures* in the approximately 6–10% of patients who demonstrate a positive acute vasodilator response,[83–85] and this is associated with very significant improvements in both symptoms and survival in this small subset of patients. Most calcium antagonists, however, with the possible exception of amlodipine,[86] are contraindicated in patients who have developed significant right ventricular dysfunction secondary to PAH, because of their negative inotropic effects.[87] The clinical conundrum relating to the use of calcium antagonists in the context of advanced PAH highlights the need for specialist management and continuous monitoring.

Prostacyclin (PGI₂) analogues

Prostacyclin (or epoprostenol) was first used clinically in 1985 to bridge a patient with primary pulmonary hypertension to heart–lung transplantation and, until 2001, when bosentan (an endothelin antagonist) first became available, this remained the only definitive medical treatment for PAH.[5,76] Epoprostenol is administered by continuous intravenous infusion (the half-life is only minutes) and, this, combined with the cost, has limited its widespread use. Epoprostenol has been shown to reverse the vascular endothelial abnormalities and resulting hypercoagulable state associated with PAH.[88] It has been shown to improve quality of life, exercise capacity and survival in PAH patients with WHO functional Class III and IV symptoms[89] and delay (in some cases remove) the need for lung transplantation.[90]

---

* Such a response is defined as a fall of > 10 mmHg in mean pulmonary artery pressure (PAP) to < 40 mmHg, associated with a stable or even increased cardiac output.

In the context of the high cost, and risks of long-term continuous intravenous administration, there have been efforts to administer such therapy via inhaled, subcutaneous, and oral routes. Agents such as iloprost (inhaled) and beraprost (oral), synthetic analogues of prostacyclin, have shown clinical benefit in PAH.[18,91,92] Unfortunately, the frequency of inhalation required with iloprost therapy, and the lack of sustained response from beraprost has limited their monotherapy role in managing PAH.[91] Another PGI_2 analogue, treprostinil, is administered subcutaneously via continuous infusion. However, local toxicity (mainly pain) at the infusion site may limit the dose, and therefore effectiveness.[93] Despite their limitations, all of these agents have proven effective in clinical use, and all provide effective treatment alternatives in selected patients.[94]

Endothelin receptor antagonists

Endothelin (ET) has emerged as a key mediator in the pathogenesis of PAH. Endothelin, in addition to being a potent vasoconstrictor, has been directly associated with fibrosis (predominantly mediated via the ET_B receptor), vascular cell hypertrophy, inflammation, and neurohormonal activation. There is heightened interest in the therapeutic role of ET_A and ET_B receptor antagonists and currently three endothelin receptor antagonists are approved in various countries around the world: bosentan, ambrisentan, and sitaxsentan.

Bosentan, an oral ET_A and ET_B receptor antagonist, has been shown in a number of randomized clinical trials to improve a variety of clinical outcomes in patients with idiopathic PAH, in PAH associated with connective tissue disease, and more recently in PAH associated with congenital heart disease.[79,95–98] In two pivotal studies, bosentan was associated with highly significant improvements in 6-minute walk tests (6MWTs) and haemodynamic measures when compared with placebo.[79,97] In three further randomized placebo-controlled studies of patients in NYHA functional Class II–IV, bosentan therapy was associated with a reduction in the time to clinical worsening (death, hospitalization due to worsening PAH, lung transplant, or epoprostenol salvage therapy) or what could be called a morbidity and mortality endpoint related to PAH.[79,97,98] An echocardiographic substudy conducted within the BREATHE-I trial demonstrated improvement in right ventricular systolic function and left ventricular early diastolic filling, in addition to a reversal of right ventricular remodelling.[99] Data now suggest that bosentan may also impact positively on survival in the aforementioned patient subgroups, and recent Australian data have demonstrated significant improvements in quality of life indices in patients with idiopathic and scleroderma-associated PAH.[23,100–103]

It should be noted that dose-related liver function abnormalities were noted in all of these studies: with the abnormalities reversible with dose titration (reduction) or cessation of treatment. Recent data suggest, following a recommended monitoring algorithm, approximately 3% of patients will need to be permanently removed from therapy due to these adverse effects on hepatic function.[104]

Sitaxsentan is also an oral ET_A receptor antagonist. Sitaxsentan has demonstrated significant improvements in 6MWT and functional class in patients with idiopathic PAH, PAH associated with connective tissue disease, and a small cohort of patients with congenital heart disease (NYHA Class II and III). There was no significant change in the time to clinical worsening compared to placebo in either of two published randomized trials (STRIDE-1 and STRIDE-2).[105,106] Girgis and colleagues have shown sitaxsentan to be effective in both 6MWT and haemodynamics in a short-term study in PAH associated with a connective tissue disorder.[107] Some data suggest sitaxsentan may be an option in those patients who discontinue bosentan due to elevated liver enzymes.[108]

Similarly, ambrisentan is another oral ET_A antagonist that has recently become available to treat PAH. Ambrisentan has demonstrated significant improvements in the 6MWT and haemodynamics (mPAP and CI), and delayed the time to clinical worsening in patients with PAH (NYHA Class II–IV). In a pre-specified combined analysis of the ARIES-1 and ARIES-2 studies, ambrisentan therapy was associated with significant improvements in the 6MWT, functional class, health-related quality of life, and the Borg dyspnoea index.[109–111] Importantly, in a combined analysis of these two 12-week studies, no patients were reported to experience elevations in their liver enzymes while receiving ambrisentan.

Both of these two new endothelin receptor antagonists provide new alternatives to clinicians in the management of PAH. As such, long-term data on the relative efficacy of ambrisentan and sitaxsentan are now eagerly awaited to confirm their definitive place in the therapeutic armoury used to effectively treat PAH.

Phosphodiesterase type 5 inhibitors

Sildenafil is an oral phosphodiesterase type 5 inhibitor and has been shown to be an effective treatment for PAH. In addition to numerous favourable case reports, a 12-week randomized controlled study (SUPER-1) has been conducted in patients with PAH (NYHA functional Class I–IV) that has demonstrated significant improvements in the 6MWT and haemodynamics.[112] Perhaps due to type II error, the study failed to significantly show a reduction in the time to clinical worsening. The authors state, after up-titration to 80 mg tid of all patients

Table 5.2 Randomized clinical trials in PAH*

Treatment	Indication	Administration	Side effects	Combination?	RCTs	Regulatory approval
Eporostenol	PAH – iPAH and CTD/PAH	IV (continuous)	Sepsis and jaw pain	Bosentan	3	USA, Canada, Europe, Japan, Australia
Iloprost	PAH – iPAH, CTD/PAH, CTEPH	Inhaled (6–9 times daily)	Short acting	Bosentan	2	USA, China, Australia, Europe
Treprostinil	PAH – iPAH, CTD/PAH and CHD/PAH	SC (infusion)	Infusion site pain		2	USA, Europe, Australia
Beroprost	PAH – iPAH, CTD/PAH and CHD/PAH	PO (QID)	Flushing headache		2	Japan, Korea
Bosentan	PAH – iPAH, CTD/PAH and CHD/PAH	PO (BID)	Elevations of liver enzymes	Epoprosenol and sildenafil	5	USA, Canada, China, Malaysia, Singapore, Thailand, Australia, Europe
Sitaxsentan	PAH – iPAH and CTD/PAH	PO (QD)	Elevations of liver enzymes		2	Europe, Canada, Australia
Ambrisentan	PAH	PO (QD)	Elevations of liver enzymes		2	USA
Sildenafil	PAH	PO (TID)	Hypotension Visual/colour problems	Bosentan	2	USA, Canada, Europe, Australia

*Please see the production information and regulatory approval applicable to you.
RCTs–randomized controlled trials, IV–intravenous; SC–subcutaneous; PO–oral; BID–twice a day; TID–three times a day; QID–four times a day; QD–every day.

Table 5.3 *Surgical procedures for PAH*

Treatment	Indication	Contraindicated	Comments/references
Atrial septostomy: palliative procedure creating a safety valve that alleviates the high pressures to which the right heart is subjected in severe disease	Considered in severe pulmonary hypertension refractory to prostaglandin therapy, particularly where associated with recurrent syncope	Atrial septostomy is not indicated in the critically ill with severe right ventricular failure or in a patient with severe left ventricular failure	Atrial septostomy should only be performed by physicians with experience in performing this procedure with low morbidity and in a PAH specialist centre[120]
Thromboendarterectomy: surgical removal of organized thrombotic material is achieved with the stripping away of pulmonary arterial endothelium, commencing proximally in the arteries and main pulmonary extending out to segmental arteries	Recommended for all age groups. Valvular disease. Coronary artery disease	Significant lung disease is contraindicated (FEV1 30% predicted). Patients with ventriculoatrial shunts for hydrocephalus are contraindicated as they may develop distal embolic disease	The prognosis for patients with thromboembolic pulmonary hypertension is poor, with a 5-year survival of 10%[123]

(Continued)

Table 5.3 (Continued)

Treatment	Indication	Contraindicated	Comments/references
Lung and heart–lung transplantation	PAH with symptomatic progressive disease that, despite optimal medical and/or surgical treatment, leaves the patient in WHO functional Class III/IV. The 6-min walk test (6MWT) is a useful tool in the assessment of when to list patients for transplantation. Those with a 6MWT of <400 m should be considered for transplantation	Candidates should meet the internationally agreed guidelines for lung transplantation	Transplant organs are limited and transplants are only performed in specialist centres[124–129]

FEV1 = forced expiratory volume in 1 second. 6MWT – Six minute walk test.

remaining in the open-label study, 6MWT outcomes remained stable after 12 months of therapy.[112] Several other studies are underway to assess the clinical efficacy of a number of other phosphodiesterase inhibitors and the results are also eagerly awaited to determine their definite role in treating PAH.

Combination therapy

There is significant interest in applying combination therapy (as opposed to monotherapy) with a prostacyclin analogue, endothelin receptor antagonist, or phosphodiesterase type 5 inhibitor to (once again) dramatically improve typically poor health outcomes associated with PAH.

Several randomized placebo-controlled trials are currently underway to assess the clinical efficacy of treating patients with PAH using a combination of adjunctive therapies. It is important to note that while many experts in the field of PAH consider this to be a part of their routine practice, pending the publication of these studies, the true cost–benefits of such an approach (i.e. combination vs monotherapy) are yet to be firmly established from an evidence-based perspective. Table 5.2 shows the current number of randomized trial to support expert clinical guidelines.

Non-medical management

There are several non-medical options available for the management of severe pulmonary hypertension – see Table 5.3. These may be generic therapies for pulmonary hypertension, such as atrial septostomy,[113] or they may be specific for certain subgroups, such as pulmonary endarterectomy for patients with chronic thromboembolic pulmonary hypertension (CTPH).[114–117] Transplantation of the lungs or heart and lungs remains an option for suitable patients with any form of pulmonary hypertension, when other therapies prove ineffective.[114–123]

Summary

The evidence for effective therapy improving the survival and quality of life of patients with pulmonary hypertension is compelling. Treatment is likely to be most effective if applied earlier in the course of the disease and, given the complexity of these patients and the treatments involved, this condition is best treated by experienced clinicians at centres with experience in all aspects of diagnostic assessment and management.

Screening and management of pulmonary arterial hypertension

6

Introduction to screening and detection

The traditional view of PAH has been that of a rare, insidious, and deadly condition, most commonly afflicting young women, and unlikely to appear on the radar of the average clinician. One of the major purposes of this clinician's guide to PAH is to provide an impetus to improved recognition of this condition, by highlighting the factors given in Box 6.1.

Box 6.1   Recognition of PAH

- PAH is almost certainly more common than most studies from specialist centres would suggest

- Most cases of PAH are only diagnosed in the advanced stages of the disease process and the prognosis thereafter is extremely poor

- There are certain 'high-risk' individuals who should be monitored for PAH, and other individuals who exhibit suspicious clinical signs and symptoms who should be assessed for the possibility of underlying PAH

- Modern-day treatments offer real survival benefits to those patients with PAH fortunate enough to be accurately diagnosed and appropriately assessed and treated

- The combination of early detection and treatment of PAH with effective, more widely available treatments is likely to have a dramatic effect on the prognosis and overall impact of this condition.

The key to better outcomes for patients with PAH lies not with specialist referral centres and so-called Centres of Excellence but with those clinicians who first come into contact with patients who may be exhibiting the first signs of

PAH and/or right ventricular dysfunction. Such patients need to be adequately investigated and, if there is a strong suspicion of PAH or a confirmed diagnosis, referred to the nearest specialist centre for management.[1] This chapter outlines the most effective strategies to ensure that patients who develop PAH are recognized and then rapidly access appropriate specialist care.

High-risk patient cohorts

The latest diagnostic classification system for pulmonary hypertension provides a clear indication of those at increased risk of developing PAH.[1] These patients need careful monitoring to ensure that PAH is detected early. Factors/conditions strongly associated (if not causally) with the development of PAH are given in Box 6.2.

Box 6.2   High-risk candidates for PAH

- congenital heart disease associated with systemic-to-pulmonary shunts (e.g. Eisenmenger's syndrome)

- familial history of PAH

- acquired human immunodeficiency virus (HIV) infection

- portal hypertension/hepatic disease

- collagen vascular disease (particularly scleroderma and systemic lupus erythematosus (SLE))

- anorexic agents/toxic drugs known to be associated with the development of PAH.[67]

In addition, epidemiological studies clearly show that women are more at risk than men of developing PAH (ratio of approximately 2:1).[15] Other 'at-risk' groups who should be considered for a diagnosis of pulmonary hypertension include any patient (especially younger individuals) with unexplained dyspnoea on exertion, or disproportionately low gas transfer (DLCO).

Given the time involved, and range of diagnostic investigations required to accurately diagnose PAH, it is impractical to screen every patient for PAH. The key is to utilize the background information contained throughout this clinician's guide to recognize those at risk, and detect the presence of PAH,

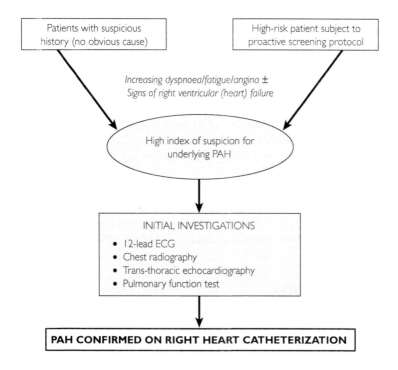

Figure 6.1 Algorithm for detecting PAH.

prompting further investigation. For those patients most at risk of developing PAH (e.g. those with scleroderma), this means regular review and specific interrogation for typical signs and symptoms. For example, Proudman and colleagues recommend a specific assessment pathway for detecting lung disease in patients with connective tissue disease.[59]

Detecting PAH

Figure 6.1 shows the various detection pathways that can be used to determine the potential of PAH and how this might lead to its definitive diagnosis through a logical series of investigations.

In addition, 'incidental' detection of PAH should not be underestimated. For example, a patient with vague symptoms and a fairly innocuous clinical profile may surprise the clinician with an electrocardiogram (ECG) similar to that shown in Figure 4.2. Such a patient then requires more intensive investigation (e.g. exercise echocardiography[70]) to determine any underlying pathology, remembering that exertional dyspnoea is the most common presenting symptom.

It follows then that the number of incidental detections of PAH could be increased if more clinicians were aware of PAH and considered it in the differential diagnosis, particularly of patients in the previously mentioned increased risk categories.

Specialist clinicians in fields outside of the PAH Centres of Excellence have an equally important role in identifying patients who would benefit from early identification and treatment. These fields include rheumatology, respiratory medicine, general cardiology, and immunology, at both consultant specialist and registrar levels.

Diagnosing PAH

Currently, the definitive diagnosis of PH of any form is achieved by right heart catheterization and direct measurement of cardiopulmonary haemodynamics. PAH, per se, is then diagnosed by excluding raised pulmonary venous/left atrial pressure (most commonly by finding a normal pulmonary capillary wedge pressure).[66,68] Other cardiopulmonary pathology that causes exertional dyspnoea can be excluded using non-invasive means (e.g. pulmonary function tests, high-resolution CT scanning and echocardiography). Recent studies indicate a potential role for selective screening with brain natriuretic peptides, which increase in the presence of elevated ventricular filling pressures secondary to PAH, to increase PAH detection rates and may be used as an adjunctive therapeutic marker for the success or failure of applied treatment strategies.[130] However, detecting patients in the latter stages of the natural history of PAH is clearly suboptimal.

Figure 6.2 is a 'diagnostic pathway' that shows how the two most important screening tests for PAH – transthoracic echocardiography and pulmonary function test – can be used to filter patients towards more definitive treatment and diagnosis (i.e. irrespective of whether a definitive diagnosis of PAH is made).

Given that there are different forms of PAH and many other causes of pulmonary hypertension per se (e.g. left-sided heart failure or valvular disease,

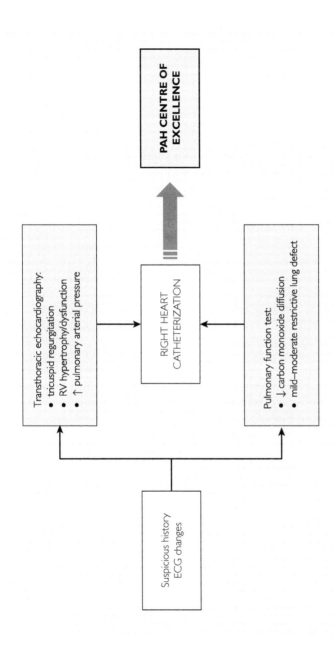

Figure 6.2 Algorithm for diagnosing PAH.

45

and thromboembolic disease), there are a number of additional investigations that may be required. These include:

- ventilation perfusion scan
- high-resolution CT
- CT or magnetic resonance pulmonary angiogram
- sleep studies.

These assessments are best undertaken at a specialist centre, with physicians experienced in the diagnosis and management of the whole range of conditions associated with pulmonary hypertension.

A new era of PAH management

Although the importance of the PAH Centres of Excellence should not be understated, with the new era of effective agents available many more clinicians now have a sound reason to increase their levels of suspicion for PAH and diagnose this condition, particularly in those patients presenting with shortness of breath and/or fatigue of unknown origin. The emergence of new oral agents such as the endothelin receptor antagonists, new forms of pre-existing therapy (e.g. oral prostacyclin analogues) and, potentially, completely new treatment options (e.g. phosphodiesterase 5 type inhibitors), particularly when combined, enables clinicians to abandon the therapeutic nihilism of past decades and offer patients effective therapies. Some of these agents allow reverse remodelling of the right ventricle and the potential to reverse the entire disease process.

APPENDIX
Informative websites: pulmonary arterial hypertension

http://www.pha-uk.com/
The Pulmonary Hypertension Association (UK) aims to provide support, understanding, and information for all those people whose lives are touched by pulmonary hypertension.

http://www.pphcure.org/
The PPH Cure Foundation (USA) provides information for the public and families affected by PPH. It is also the world's largest non-government foundation providing funding for PPH research.

http://www.phassociation.org/
A public website, providing news and research updates on pulmonary hypertension (USA), that is dedicated to increasing advocacy and awareness of pulmonary hypertension.

http://www.phcentral.org/
The PHCentral (USA) mission is to be the definitive internet resource for pulmonary hypertension-related information for patients, caregivers, and medical professionals.

http://www.mayoclinic.org/pulmonaryhypertension-rst/
Public information about the treatment of pulmonary hypertension at the Mayo Clinic (USA).

http://www.pah-info.com
Actelion, the makers of bosentan (Tracleer), provides information on pulmonary arterial hypertension for health care professionals and consumers, including links to global patient networks.

http://www.pah.com.au
Actelion, the makers of bosentan (Tracleer), provides information on pulmonary arterial hypertension for Australian health care professionals as well as consumers.

http://www.actelion.com/
Actelion, the makers of bosentan, provides pharmaceutical information and research on drug trials (Swiss).

http://www.gilead.com/
Gilead is the marketer of ambrisentan in the USA.

http://www.pfizer.com/home/
Pfizer is the marketer of Revatio (sildenafil).

http://www.encysive.com/
Encysive Pharmaceuticals is the marketer of sitaxsentan.

http://www.gsk.com/
GlaxoSmithKline is the marketer of Flolan (epoprostenol).

http://www.scleroderma.org/
The Scleroderma Foundation (USA) provides public information, education research, and chat room facilities for patients and families seeking contact and support. It includes links to other related sites.

http://www.lupusnsw.org.au/ie.html
The Lupus Association of NSW Inc. (Australia) is a community-based counselling and advocacy service with over 1100 members throughout New South Wales and Australian Capital Territory, and a permanently staffed office at North Ryde in Sydney, New South Wales.

http://www.unither.com/
United Therapeutics, the makers of tresprostinil (Remodulin), provides information about prostacyclins.

http://www.sclerodermaaustralia.com.au
This website has been created to support the scleroderma community in Australia. It provides information about the disease, medical services, and research into scleroderma.

http://www.mja.com.au/public/issues/178_11_020603/keo10709_fm.pdf
Clinical update from Dr Anne Keogh and team from the *Medical Journal of Australia*.

http://www.ishlt.org/
The International Society for Heart & Lung Transplantation.

References

1. Simmoneau G, Nazzareno G, Rubin LJ et al. Clinical classification of pulmonary hypertension. J Am Coll Cardiol 2004; 43(Suppl S): 5S–12S.
2. Rich S (ed.). World Health Organisation: primary pulmonary hypertension – executive summary, World Symposium, Primary Pulmonary Hypertension 1998. Available at: http://www.who.int/ncd/cvd/pph.html (accessed Nov 2003).
3. Keogh AM, McNeil KD, Williams T et al. Pulmonary arterial hypertension: a new era in management. MJA 2003; 178: 564–7.
4. Rich S, Dantzker DR, Ayers SM et al. Primary pulmonary hypertension. A national prospective study. Ann Intern Med 1987; 107: 216–23.
5. D'Alonzo GE, Barst RJ, Ayers SM et al. Survival in patients with primary pulmonary hypertension. Results from a national prospective registry. Ann Intern Med 1991; 115: 343–9.
6. Koh ET, Lee P, Gladman DD, Abu-Shakra M. Pulmonary hypertension in systemic sclerosis: an analysis of 17 patients. Br J Rheum 1996; 35: 989–93.
7. Preston IR, Hill NS. Evaluation and management of pulmonary hypertension in systemic sclerosis. Curr Opin Rheumatol 2003; 15: 761–5.
8. Denton CP, Black CM. Pulmonary hypertension in systemic sclerosis. Rheum Dis Clin North Am 2003; 29: 335–49.
9. Humbert M, Sitbon O, Chaouat A et al. Pulmonary arterial hypertension in France. Am J Resp Crit Care Med 2006; 173: 1023–30.
10. Carrington M, Murphy NF, Strange G et al. Prognostic impact of pulmonary arterial hypertension: a population based analysis. Int J Cardiol 2007 Apr 10; [Epub ahead of print]
11. Abenhaim L, Moride Y, Brenot F et al. Appetite suppressant drugs and the risk of primary pulmonary hypertension. International Primary Pulmonary Hypertension Study Group. N Engl J Med 1996; 335: 609–16.
12. Hallioglu O, Dilber E, Celiker A. Comparison of acute hemodynamic effects of aerosolized and intravenous iloprost in secondary pulmonary hypertension in children with congenital heart disease. Am J Cardiol 2003; 92: 1007–9.
13. Zuber JP, Calmy A, Evison JM et al. Pulmonary arterial hypertension related to HIV infection: improved hemodynamics and survival associated with antiretroviral therapy. Clin Infect Dis 2004; 38: 1178–85.

14. Benjaminov FS, Prentice M, Sniderman KW et al. Portopulmonary hypertension in decompensated cirrhosis with refractory ascites. Gut 2003; 52: 1355–62.

15. Peacock AJ, Murphy NF, McMurray JJ, Caballero L, Stewart S. An epidemiological study of pulmonary arterial hypertension in Scotland. Eur Respir J 2007; 30: 104–9.

16. Galiè N, Torbicki A, Barst R et al; Task Force. Guidelines on diagnosis and treatment of pulmonary arterial hypertension. The Task Force on Diagnosis and Treatment of Pulmonary Arterial Hypertension of the European Society of Cardiology. Eur Heart J 2004; 25(24): 2243–78.

17. Rubin LJ; American College of Chest Physicians. Diagnosis and management of pulmonary arterial hypertension: ACCP evidence-based clinical practice guidelines. Chest 2004; 126(1 Suppl): 4S–6S.

18. Badesch DB, Abman SH, Simonneau G, Rubin LJ, McLaughlin VV. Medical therapy for pulmonary arterial hypertension: updated ACCP evidence-based clinical practice guidelines. Chest 2007; 131(6): 1917–28.

19. Perloff JK, Hart EM, Greaves SM et al. Proximal pulmonary arterial and intra-pulmonary radiologic features of Eisenmenger syndrome and primary pulmonary hypertension. Am J Cardiol 2003; 92: 182–7.

20. Granton JT, Rabinovitch M. Pulmonary arterial hypertension in congenital heart disease. Cardiol Clin 2002; 20: 441–57.

21. Nakamura M, Yoshida H, Naganuma Y et al. Peripheral vasodilatory dysfunction in adult patients with congenital heart disease and severely elevated pulmonary vascular resistance. Angiology 2002; 53: 715–20.

22. Kendrick S, Clarke J. The Scottish record linkage system. Health Bull 1993; 51: 72–9.

23. Williams MH, Das C, Handler CE et al. Systemic sclerosis associated pulmonary hypertension: improved survival in the current era. Heart 2006; 92: 926–32.

24. Hubert M, Morrell NW, Archer SL et al. Cellular and molecular pathobiology of pulmonary arterial hypertension. J Am Coll Cardiol 2004; 43: S13–24.

25. Bolster MA, Hogan J, Bredin CP. Pulmonary vascular occlusive disease presenting as sudden death. Med Sci Law 1990; 30: 26–8.

26. Paakko P, Sutinen S, Remes M et al. A case of pulmonary vascular occlusive disease: comparison of post-mortem radiography and histology. Histopathology 1985; 9: 253–62.

27. Galiè N, Manes A, Uguccioni L et al. Primary pulmonary hypertension: insights into pathogenesis from epidemiology. Chest 1998; 114: 184–94S.

28. Palevsky HI, Schloo BL, Pietra GG et al. Primary pulmonary hypertension. Vascular structure, morphometry and responsiveness to vascular agents. Circulation 1989; 80: 1207–21.

29. Rubin LJ. Therapy of pulmonary hypertension: the evolution from vasodilators to antiproliferative agents. Am J Respir Crit Care Med 2002; 166: 1308–9.

30. McLaughlin VV, McGoon MD. Pulmonary arterial hypertension. Circulation 2006; 114(13): 1417–31.
31. Altman R, Scazziota A, Rouvier J et al. Coagulation and fibrinolytic parameters in patients with pulmonary hypertension. Chest 1996; 19: 549–54.
32. Welsh CH, Hassel KL, Badesch DB et al. Coagulation and fibrinolytic profiles in patients with severe pulmonary hypertension. Chest 1996; 110: 710–17.
33. Kamata S, Kamiyama M, Usui N et al. Is adrenomedullin involved in the pathophysiology of persistent pulmonary hypertension of the newborn? Pediatr Surg Int 2004; 20: 24–6.
34. Ono F, Nagaya N, Okamura H et al. Effect of orally active prostacyclin analogue on survival in patients with chronic thromboembolic pulmonary hypertension without major vessel obstruction. Chest 2003; 123: 1583–8.
35. Galie N, Manes A, Branzi A. Emerging medical therapies for pulmonary arterial hypertension. Prog Cardiov Dis 2003; 45: 213–24.
36. Nagaya N, Sasaki N, Ando M et al. Prostacyclin therapy before pulmonary thromboendarterectomy in patients with chronic thromboembolic pulmonary hypertension. Chest 2003; 123: 338–43.
37. Channick RN, Rubin LJ. New and experimental therapies for pulmonary hypertension. Clin Chest Med 2001; 3: 539–45.
38. Yanagisawa M, Kurihara H, Kimura S et al. A novel potent vasoconstrictor peptide produced by vascular endothelial cells. Nature 1988; 332: 411–15.
39. Kim NHS, Rubin LJ. Endothelin in health and disease: endothelin receptor antagonists in the management of pulmonary arterial hypertension. J Cardiovasc Pharmacol Therapeut 2002; 7: 9–19.
40. Levin ER, Epstein FH (eds). Mechanisms of disease: endothelins. N Engl J Med 1995; 333: 356–63.
41. Roux S, Breu V, Ertel SI, Clozel M. Endothelin antagonism with bosentan: a review of potential applications. J Mol Med 1999; 77: 364–76.
42. Giaid A, Yanagisawa M, Langleben D et al. Expression of endothelin-1 in the lungs of patients with pulmonary hypertension. N Engl J Med 1993; 328: 1732–9.
43. Galiè N, Grigioni F, Bacchi-Reggiani L et al. Relation of endothelin-1 to survival in patients with primary pulmonary hypertension. Eur J Clin Invest 1996; 26: 273.
44. Clozel M, Gray GA, Breu V et al. The endothelin ET B receptor mediates both vasodilation and vasoconstriction in vivo. Biochem Biophys Res Commun 1992; 186(2): 867–73.
45. Sullivan CC, Du L, Chu D et al. Induction of pulmonary hypertension by an angiopoietin 1/TIE2/serotonin pathway. Proc Natl Acad Sci USA 2003; 100: 12331–66.
46. Yun S, Junbao D, Limin G et al. The regulating effect of heme oxygenase/carbon monoxide on hypoxic pulmonary vascular structural remodeling. Biochem Biophys Res Commun 2003; 306: 523–9.

47. Runo JR, Lloyd JE. Primary pulmonary hypertension. Lancet 2003; 361: 1533–44.

48. Yamane K. Endothelin and collagen vascular disease: a review with special reference to Raynaud's phenomenon and systemic sclerosis. Intern Med 1994; 33: 579–82.

49. Hoeper MM. Sitaxsentan in pulmonary arterial hypertension: a viewpoint of Marious M Hoeper. Drugs 2007; 67(5): 771–2.

50. Barst RJ. A review of pulmonary hypertension: role of ambrisentan. Vasc Health Risk Manag 2007; 3(1): 11–22.

51. Hartness ME, Brazier SP, Peers C et al. Post-transcriptional control of human maxiK potassium channel activity and acute oxygen sensitivity by chronic hypoxia. J Biol Chem 2003; 278: 51422–32.

52. Mandegar M, Remillard CV, Yuan JX. Ion channels in pulmonary arterial hypertension. Prog Cardiovasc Dis 2002; 45: 81–114.

53. Mandegar M, Yuan JX. Role of K^+ channels in pulmonary hypertension. Vasc Pharmacol 2002; 38: 25–33.

54. Lloyd JE, Butler MG, Foroud TM et al. Genetic anticipation and abnormal gender ratio at birth in familial primary pulmonary hypertension. Am J Respir Crit Care Med 1995; 152: 93–7.

55. West J, Fagan K, Steudel W et al. Pulmonary hypertension in transgenic mice expressing a dominant-negative BMPRII gene in smooth muscle. Circ Res 2004; 94: 1109–14.

56. Thomson JR, Machado RD, Pauciulo MW et al. Sporadic primary pulmonary hypertension is associated with germline mutations in BMPR2, a receptor member of the TGF-beta family. J Med Genet 2000; 37: 741–5.

57. Du L, Sullivan CC, Chu D et al. Signaling molecules in nonfamilial pulmonary hypertension. N Engl J Med 2003; 348: 500–9.

58. Gurtner HP. Aminorex and pulmonary hypertension. A review. Cor Vasa 1995; 27: 160–71.

59. Proudman SM, Stevens WM, Sahhar J, Celermajer D. Pulmonary arterial hypertension in systemic sclerosis: the need for early detection and treatment. Intern Med J 2007; 37(7): 485–94.

60. Barbarinia G, Barbaro G. Incidence of the involvement of the cardiovascular system in HIV infection. AIDS 2003; 17(Suppl 1): S46–50.

61. Egito ES, Aiello VD, Bosisio IB et al. Vascular remodeling process in reversibility of pulmonary arterial hypertension secondary to congenital heart disease. Pathol Res Pract 2003; 199: 521–32.

62. MacGregor AJ, Canavan R, Knight C et al. Pulmonary hypertension in systemic sclerosis: risk factors for progression and consequences for survival. Rheumatology 2001; 40: 453–9.

63. Fuster V, Steele PM, Edwards WD et al. Primary pulmonary hypertension: natural history and the importance of thrombosis. Circulation 1984; 70: 580–7.

64. Kanemoto N. Natural history of pulmonary hemodynamics in primary pulmonary hypertension. Am Heart J 1987; 114: 407–13.
65. Eysmann SB, Palevsky HI, Reichek N et al. Two-dimensional and Doppler-echocardiographic and cardiac correlates of survival in primary pulmonary hypertension. Circulation 1989; 80: 353–60.
66. Barst RJ, McGoon M, Torbicki A et al. Diagnosis and differential assessment of pulmonary arterial hypertension. J Am Coll Cardiol 2004; 43(Suppl S): 40–47S.
67. Denton CP, Cailes JB, Phillips GD et al. Comparison of Doppler echocardiography and right heart catheterisation to assess pulmonary hypertension in systemic sclerosis. Br J Rheum 1997; 36: 239–43.
68. Yock P, Popp R. Noninvasive estimation of right ventricular systolic pressure by Doppler ultrasound in patients with tricuspid regurgitation. Circulation 1994; 70: 657.
69. Mukerjee D, St George D, Knight C et al. Echocardiography and pulmonary function as screening tests for pulmonary arterial hypertension in systemic sclerosis. Rheumatology 2004; 43: 461–6.
70. Collins N, Bastian B, Quiqueree L et al. Abnormal pulmonary vascular responses in patients registered with a systemic autoimmunity database: Pulmonary Hypertension Assessment and Screening Evaluation using stress echocardiography (PHASE-I). Eur J Echocardiogr 2006; 7(6): 439–46.
71. The New York Heart Association. Diseases of the heart and blood vessels; nomenclature and criteria for diagnosis, 6th edn. Boston: Little Brown and Co., 1964.
72. Fletcher GF, Baladay G, Froelicher VF et al. Exercise standards: a statement for healthcare professionals from the American Heart Association writing group. Circulation 1995; 91: 580–615.
73. Enright PL, Sherrill DL. Reference equations for the six-minute walk in healthy adults. Am J Respir Crit Care Med 1998; 158: 1384–7.
74. Bittner V, Weiner DH, Yusuf S et al. Prediction of mortality and morbidity with a 6-minute walk test in patients with left ventricular dysfunction. JAMA 1993; 270: 1702–7.
75. Miyamoto S, Nagaya N, Satoh T et al. Clinical correlates and prognostic significance of six-minute walk test in patients with primary pulmonary hypertension. Am J Respir Crit Care Med 2000; 161: 487–92.
76. Nazzareno G, Seeger W, Naeije R et al. Comparative analysis of clinical trials and evidence-based treatment algorithm in pulmonary arterial hypertension. J Am Coll Cardiol 2004; 43(Suppl S): S76–88.
77. Kim NH, Channick RN, Rubin LJ. Successful withdrawal of long-term epoprostenol therapy for pulmonary arterial hypertension. Chest 2003; 124: 1612–15.
78. Sitbon O, McLaughlin V, Badesch D et al. Comparison of two treatment strategies, first-line bosentan or epoprostenol on survival in Class III idiopathic pulmonary arterial hypertension. Am J Crit Care Med 2004; 169(Suppl A): A210.

79. Rubin LJ, Badesch DB, Barst R et al. Bosentan therapy for pulmonary arterial hypertension. N Engl J Med 2002; 346: 896–903.
80. Olschewski H, Simonneau G, Galiè N et al. Inhaled iloprost for severe pulmonary hypertension. N Engl J Med 2002; 347: 322–9.
81. Galiè N, Ghofrani HA, Torbicki A et al. Sildenafil Use in Pulmonary Arterial Hypertension (SUPER) Study Group. Sildenafil citrate therapy for pulmonary arterial hypertension. N Engl J Med 2005; 353(20): 2148–57.
82. Rich S, Seiditz M, Dodin E. The short-term effects of digoxin in patients with right ventricular dysfunction from pulmonary hypertension. Chest 1998; 114: 787–92.
83. Rich S, Kauffman E, Levy PS. The effects of high dose calcium-channel blockers on the survival in primary pulmonary hypertension. N Engl J Med 1992; 327: 76–81.
84. Sitbon O, Humbert M, Ioos V et al. Who benefits from long-term calcium-channel blocker (CCB) therapy in primary pulmonary hypertension (PPH). Am J Crit Care 2003; 167: A440.
85. Morales-Blanhir J, Santos S, de Jover L et al. Clinical value of vasodilator test with inhaled nitric oxide for predicting long-term response to oral vasodilators in pulmonary hypertension. Respir Med 2004; 98: 225–34.
86. Packer M, O'Connor CM, Ghali JK. Effect of amlodipine on morbidity and mortality in severe chronic heart failure. Prospective Randomised Amlodipine Survival Evaluation Study Group. N Engl J Med 1996; 335: 1107–14.
87. Mehra MR, Uber PA, Francis GA. Heart failure therapy at a crossroad: are there limits to the neurohormonal model? J Am Coll Cardiol 2003; 41: 1606–10.
88. Clapp LH, Finney P, Turcato S et al. Differential effects of stable prostacyclin analogs on smooth muscle proliferation and cyclic AMP generation in human pulmonary artery. Am J Respir Cell Mol Biol 2002; 2: 194–201.
89. McLaughlin VV, Shillington A, Rich S. Survival in primary pulmonary hypertension: the impact of epoprostenol therapy. Circulation 2002; 106: 1477–82.
90. Barst RJ, Rubin LJ, Long WA et al. A comparison of continuous intravenous epoprostenol (prostacyclin) with conventional therapy for primary pulmonary hypertension. The Primary Pulmonary Hypertension Study Group. N Engl J Med 1996; 334(5): 296–302.
91. Barst RJ, McGoon M, McLaughlin V et al. Beraprost Study Group. Beraprost therapy for pulmonary arterial hypertension. J Am Coll Cardiol 2003; 41(12): 2119–25.
92. De Wet CJ, Affleck DG, Jacobsohn E et al. Inhaled prostacyclin is safe, effective, and affordable in patients with pulmonary hypertension, right heart dysfunction, and refractory hypoxemia after cardiothoracic surgery. J Thorac Cardiovasc Surg 2004; 127: 1058–67.
93. Strauss WL, Edelman JD. Prostanoid therapy for pulmonary arterial hypertension. Clin Chest Med 2007; 28(1): 127–42.

94. Simonneau G, Barst RJ, Galie N et al; Treprostinil Study Group. Continuous subcutaneous infusion of treprostinil, a prostacyclin analogue, in patients with pulmonary arterial hypertension: a double-blind, randomized, placebo-controlled trial. Am J Respir Crit Care Med 2002; 165(6): 800–4.

95. Galie N, Beghetti M, Gatzoulis MA et al; Bosentan Randomized Trial of Endothelin Antagonist Therapy-5 (BREATHE-5) Investigators. Bosentan therapy in patients with Eisenmenger syndrome: a multicenter, double-blind, randomized, placebo-controlled study. Circulation 2006; 114(1): 48–54.

96. Gatzoulis MA, Beghetti M, Galie N et al; on behalf of the BREATHE-5 Investigators. Longer-term bosentan therapy improves functional capacity in Eisenmenger syndrome: results of the BREATHE-5 open-label extension study. Int J Cardiol 2007 Jul 19; [Epub ahead of print]

97. Channick RN, Simonneau G, Sitbon O et al; Effects of the dual endothelin-receptor antagonist bosentan in patients with pulmonary hypertension: a randomised placebo-controlled study. Lancet 2001; 358: 1119–23.

98. Galie N, Rubin L, Heoper M et al. Bosentan improves hemodynamics and delays time to clinical worsening in patients with mildly symptomatic pulmonary arterial hypertension (PAH): results of the EARLY study. Eur Heart J 2007; 28(abstract supplement): 140.

99. Galie N, Hinderliter AL, Torbicki A et al. Effects of the oral endothelin-receptor antagonist bosentan on echocardiographic and Doppler measures in patients with pulmonary arterial hypertension. J Am Coll Cardiol 2003; 41: 1380–6.

100. McLaughlin VV. Survival in patients with pulmonary arterial hypertension treated with first-line bosentan. Eur J Clin Invest 2006; 36(Suppl 3): 10–15.

101. Keogh AM, McNeil KD, Wlodarczyk J, Gabbay E, Williams TJ. Quality of life in pulmonary arterial hypertension: improvement and maintenance with bosentan. J Heart Lung Transplant 2007; 26(2): 181–7.

102. Denton CP, Humbert M, Rubin L, Black CM. Bosentan treatment for pulmonary arterial hypertension related to connective tissue disease: a subgroup analysis of the pivotal clinical trials and their open-label extensions. Ann Rheum Dis 2006; 65(10): 1336–40.

103. Provencher S, Sitbon O, Humbert M et al. Long-term outcome with first-line bosentan therapy in idiopathic pulmonary arterial hypertension. Eur Heart J 2006; 27(5): 589–95.

104. Humbert M, Segal ES, Kiely DG et al. Results of European post-marketing surveillance of bosentan in pulmonary hypertension. Eur Respir J 2007; 30(2): 338–44.

105. Langleben D, Brock T, Dixon R, Barst R; STRIDE-1 study group. STRIDE 1: Effects of the selective ETA receptor antagonist, sitaxsentan sodium, in a patient population with pulmonary arterial hypertension that meets traditional inclusion criteria of previous pulmonary arterial hypertension trials. J Cardiovasc Pharmacol 2004; 44: S80–4.

106. Barst RJ, Langleben D, Badesch D et al; STRIDE-2 Study Group. Treatment of pulmonary arterial hypertension with the selective endothelin-A receptor antagonist sitaxsentan. J Am Coll Cardiol 2006; 47(10): 2049–56.

107. Girgis RE, Frost AE, Hill NS et al. Selective endothelinA receptor antagonism with sitaxsentan for pulmonary arterial hypertension associated with connective tissue disease. Ann Rheum Dis 2007; 66(11): 1467–72.

108. Benza RL, Mehta S, Keogh A et al. Sitaxsentan treatment for patients with pulmonary arterial hypertension discontinuing bosentan. J Heart Lung Transplant 2007; 26(1): 63–9.

109. Galié N, Badesch D, Oudiz R et al. Ambrisentan therapy for pulmonary arterial hypertension. J Am Coll Cardiol 2005; 46(3): 529–35.

110. Olschewski H, Galie N, Kramer M et al. Ambrisentan improves exercise capacity and time to clinical worsening in patients with pulmonary arterial hypertension: Results of the ARIES-2 study. Am J Respir Crit Care Med 2006; Suppl A: A728(Abstract).

111. Galie N, Olschewski H, Rubin L, the ARIES study group. Ambrisentan therapy for pulmonary arterial hypertension: an intergrated analysis of the ARIES-1 and ARIES-2 studies. Am J Respir Crit Care Med 2007; Suppl A: A397(Abstract).

112. Galiè N, Ghofrani HA, Torbicki A et al. Sildenafil Use in Pulmonary Arterial Hypertension (SUPER) Study Group. Sildenafil citrate therapy for pulmonary arterial hypertension. N Engl J Med 2005; 353(20): 2148–57.

113. Rich S, Dodin E, McLaughlin V. Usefulness of atrial septostomy as a treatment for primary pulmonary hypertension and guidelines for its application. Am J Cardiol 1997; 80: 369–71.

114. Keck BM, Bennett LE, Rosendale J et al. Worldwide thoracic organ transplantation: a report from UNOS/ISHLT International Registry for Thoracic Organ Transplantation. Clin Transpl 1998; 39–52.

115. Jamieson SW. Pulmonary thromboendarterectomy. Heart 1998; 79: 118–20.

116. Mayer E, Dahm M, Hake U et al. Mid-term results of pulmonary thromboendarterectomy for chronic thromboembolic pulmonary hypertension. Ann Thorac Surg 1996; 61: 1788–92.

117. Moser KM, Auger WR, Fedullo PF et al. Chronic thromboembolic pulmonary hypertension: clinical picture and surgical treatment. Eur Respir J 1992; 5: 334–42.

118. Reitz BA, Wallwork JL, Hunt SA et al. Heart–lung transplantation: successful therapy for patients with pulmonary vascular disease. N Engl J Med 1982; 306: 557–64.

119. Pasque MK, Kaiser LR, Dresler CM et al. Single lung transplantation for pulmonary hypertension. Technical aspects and immediate haemodynamic results. J Thorac Cardiovasc Surg 1992; 103: 475–81.

120. Pasque MK, Cooper JD, Kaiser LR et al. Improved technique for bilateral lung transplantation: rationale and initial clinical experience. Ann Thorac Surg 1990; 49: 785–91.

121. Meyers BF, Lynch J, Trulock EP, et al. Lung transplantation: a decade of experience. Ann Surg 1999; 230: 362–70.

122. The American Society for Transplant Physicians (ASTP)/The American Thoracic Society (ATS)/European Respiratory Society (ERS)/International Society for Heart Lung Transplantation (ISHLT). International guidelines for the selection of lung transplantation. Am J Respir Crit Care Med 1997; 158: 335–9.

123. Evans TW, Gatzoulis MA, Gibbs JSR. A national pulmonary hypertension service for England and Wales: an orphan disease adopted? Thorax 2002; 57: 471–2.

124. Weitzenblum E, Sautegeau A, Ehrhart M. Long-term oxygen therapy can reverse the progression of pulmonary hypertension in patients with chronic obstructive pulmonary disease. Am Rev Respir Dis 1985; 131: 493–8.

125. Royal College of Physicians Working Party. Domiciliary oxygen therapy services. London: Royal College of Physicians, 1999.

126. Bowyer JJ, Busst CM, Denison DM, Shinebourne EA. Effect of long term oxygen treatment at home in children with pulmonary vascular disease. Br Heart J 1986; 55: 385–90.

127. Turbow R, Waffarn F, Yang L et al. Variable oxygenation response to inhaled nitric oxide in severe persistent pulmonary hypertension of the newborn. Acta Paediatr 1995; 84: 1305–8.

128. Remme WJ, Swedberg K. Guidelines for the diagnosis and treatment of chronic heart failure. Eur Heart J 2001; 22: 1527–60.

129. Rich S, Seiditz M, Dodin E. The short term effects of digoxin in patients with right ventricular dysfunction from pulmonary hypertension. Chest 1998; 114: 787–92.

130. Mukerjee D, Yap LB, Holmes AM et al. Significance of plasma N-terminal pro-brain natriuretic peptide in patients with systemic sclerosis-related pulmonary arterial hypertension. Respir Med 2003; 97: 1230–6.

Index

Page numbers in *italic* denote figures, tables or boxes.
PAH = pulmonary arterial hypertension

T - #1078 - 101024 - C70 - 186/123/3 - PB - 9781841846651 - Gloss Lamination